Sniffing Away Anxiety:
The Power of Body Odour as an Anxiety Therapy

By

Martha B.Kimble

Table of content

Chapter 1: Introduction

Chapter 2: Body odour Science

  The relationship between body odour and emotion

Chapter 3: Body odour Therapy for Anxiety

  Aromatherapy

  Scent Blends to Order

Chapter 4: The Advantages and Drawbacks of Body Odour Therapy for Anxiety

  Body Odour Therapy for Anxiety: Limitations

Chapter 5: Including Body Odour Therapy in Your Wellness Routine

Chapter 6: Selecting the Best Scent

Chapter 7: Body Odour Therapy Risks and Precautions

Chapter 8: Conclusion

  Resources for further information on body odour therapy

Chapter 1: Introduction

Anxiety is a common mental health problem that affects millions of people around the world. It can be a crippling condition that affects all aspects of a person's life, including work, relationships, and overall well-being. While there are many anxiety treatments available, some people prefer to experiment with alternative therapies to manage their symptoms. Body odour therapy is one such therapy that has grown in popularity in recent years.

Body odour therapy uses scents and smells to help reduce anxiety and promote relaxation. While using body odour as a therapy may appear unusual, there is scientific evidence that certain scents can have a calming effect on the mind and body.

In this book, we will look at the science behind body odour therapy and how it can be used to manage anxiety. We will go over various types of body odour therapy, such as aromatherapy and custom scent blends, as well as practical tips for incorporating these techniques into your daily life. We'll also look at the risks and precautions of using body odour therapy.

Finally, the purpose of this book is to give readers a thorough understanding of the power of body odour as an anxiety therapy and how it can be used to improve overall mental health and well-being.

Understanding Anxiety and its Consequences

Anxiety is a mental health condition marked by persistent feelings of worry, fear, and apprehension. Panic attacks, social anxiety, and generalized anxiety disorder are all examples of how they can manifest.

Anxiety can have a significant impact on a person's ability to function in daily life.

Anxiety, for example, can make it difficult to focus at work or school, maintain relationships, or even leave the house.

Anxiety can have physical consequences in addition to emotional and social ones. It can result in headaches, muscle tension, and gastrointestinal issues, among other things.

Body odour as an Anxiety Treatment

Body odour therapy is the use of scents and smells to promote relaxation and anxiety reduction. The theory behind this therapy is that certain scents can cause a brain response that helps calm the mind and body.

Aromatherapy and custom scent blends are two examples of body odour therapy. Aromatherapy uses essential oils to promote relaxation, while custom scent blends are created based on a person's specific needs and preferences.

Overall, body odour therapy is a non-invasive and natural way to manage anxiety symptoms. It can be combined with other treatments, such as therapy and medication, to provide a more comprehensive approach to anxiety management.

Conclusion

We provided an overview of the book in this chapter and discussed the importance of understanding anxiety and its impact. We also looked at the role of body odour in anxiety therapy and how it can be used as an effective tool for symptom management.

In the following chapters, we will delve deeper into the science of body odour therapy, examine various types of body odour therapy techniques, and offer practical tips for incorporating these techniques into daily life. We will also go over the potential risks and precautions of using body odour therapy.

Chapter 2: Body odour Science

Body odour is an unavoidable and natural part of being human. It is produced by the body's sweat glands and is influenced by some factors, such as genetics, diet, and hygiene. While body odour is frequently associated with negative connotations, such as poor hygiene, scientific evidence suggests that it can also have a positive impact on mental health and well-being.

In this chapter, we'll look at the science behind body odour, such as how it's created, the role of bacteria in body odour, and the connection between body odour and emotions.

What Causes Body odour?
Sweat glands of two types produce body odour: eccrine glands and apocrine glands. Eccrine glands are found throughout the body and produce sweat, which is mostly made up of water and salt. This type of sweat has no odour and is primarily used to regulate body temperature.

Apocrine glands, on the other hand, are found in places where there are hair follicles, such as the armpits and groin. These glands produce a thicker, more protein- and lipid-rich sweat. This type of sweat can produce a distinct odour when it comes into contact with bacteria on the skin.

Bacterial involvement in body odour

There are two types of sweat glands in the human body:

- Eccrine
- Appcrine

Eccrine sweat glands: This are found all over the body and produce sweat that is mostly made up of water and salt. This sweat has no strong odour and is primarily used to regulate body temperature.

Apocrine sweat glands: On the other hand, are found in specific areas of the body, such as the armpits and groin, and produce sweat that is made up of water, salt, and organic compounds. These organic compounds, such as fatty acids and proteins, are broken down by bacteria on the skin's surface, resulting in the characteristic body odour associated with apocrine sweat.

The bacteria that break down these organic compounds are mostly Staphylococcus and Corynebacterium species. When these bacteria degrade the organic compounds in sweat, they produce volatile fatty acids and other compounds that give sweat its distinct odour.

Surprisingly, the bacteria on a person's skin can affect their body odour. A study, for example, discovered that people who sweated a compound called 3-methyl-2-hexenoic acid were more likely to have a certain type of bacteria on their skin than people who did not.

Overall, bacteria play an important role in body odour, and the composition of bacteria on a person's skin can influence their body odour. Understanding the science behind body odour can help inform how body odour therapy can be used to treat anxiety.

The relationship between body odour and emotion

There is evidence that body odour is related to emotions and mood. According to research, the scent of human sweat can elicit specific emotional responses in those who smell it.

One study discovered, for example, that the scent of fear-induced sweat can cause people to become more alert. On the other hand, the scent of happiness-induced sweat can elicit positive emotions and social bonding in those who smell it.

Body odour and emotion are thought to be linked because certain chemicals found in sweat can communicate emotional states. For example, researchers discovered androstadienone in male sweat, which is thought to have a pheromone-like effect on women, eliciting a positive mood and sexual attraction.

These findings imply that body odour can be an effective tool for coping with emotions such as anxiety. It may be possible to elicit emotional responses that promote relaxation and reduce anxiety by using specific scents and odours.

Aromatherapy and custom scent blends, for example, can be used to harness the emotional power of scent and promote relaxation. Individuals may be able to reduce anxiety and improve their overall well-being by selecting scents associated with positive emotions, such as lavender or chamomile.

Chapter 3: Body odour Therapy for Anxiety

In this chapter, we will look at how body odour therapy can help with anxiety. This therapy makes use of scents and smells to promote relaxation and reduce anxiety. We will go over various methods for using body odour therapy, such as aromatherapy and custom scent blends.

Aromatherapy

Aromatherapy is a popular type of body-odour therapy in which essential oils are used to promote relaxation and reduce anxiety. Essential oils are plant extracts that are highly concentrated and contain natural aromatic compounds.

These compounds, when inhaled, can have a direct effect on the brain and nervous system, promoting relaxation and reducing feelings of anxiety. Lavender, chamomile, and bergamot are some of the most popular essential oils for anxiety.

Individuals can use aromatherapy for anxiety by diffusing essential oils in a room, adding them to a bath, or using them in massage therapy. Some people prefer to wear essential oils as a personal fragrance throughout the day.

Scent Blends to Order

Another type of body odour therapy is custom scent blends, which involve creating a unique scent that is tailored to an individual's preferences and needs. This can be accomplished by combining various essential oils or other natural scents to create a unique fragrance.

Individuals can work with a professional scent designer or create their blend at home to create a custom scent blend. Individuals can create a fragrance that promotes calmness and well-being by selecting scents that are known to promote relaxation and reduce anxiety, such as lavender or chamomile.

Other Techniques

There are other methods for using body odour therapy to manage anxiety besides aromatherapy and custom scent blends. To reduce body odour and promote a sense of freshness and cleanliness, some people may choose to wear clothing made of natural fibers, such as cotton or linen.

Others may prefer natural deodourants that are free of synthetic fragrances and aluminum, both of which can be irritating to the skin and potentially harmful to health.

Overall, body odour therapy can be an effective tool for anxiety management. Individuals can improve their overall well-being and quality of life by using scents and smell to promote relaxation and reduce feelings of anxiety.

Chapter 4: The Advantages and Drawbacks of Body Odour Therapy for Anxiety

In this chapter, we will look at the benefits and drawbacks of body odour therapy for anxiety management.

The Advantages of Body odour Therapy for Anxiety

One of the primary advantages of body odour therapy is that it is non-invasive and natural. Body odour therapy, unlike other forms of therapy such as medication or talk therapy, does not involve the use of synthetic chemicals or invasive procedures.

Body odour therapy is also simple to incorporate into daily routines, making it a convenient and accessible form of therapy for many people. Furthermore, body odour therapy can be tailored to individual preferences and needs, allowing people to create a scent that is tailored to their specific needs and preferences.

Another advantage of body odour therapy is its ability to promote relaxation and reduce feelings of anxiety. Certain scents and smells, such as lavender and chamomile, have been shown in studies to have a calming effect on the brain and nervous system, promoting relaxation and reducing feelings of anxiety.

Body Odour Therapy for Anxiety: Limitations

While body odour therapy can be beneficial in reducing anxiety, it is not a panacea. It may not be effective for everyone and may not be sufficient for severe cases of anxiety on its own.

Furthermore, body odour therapy may be ineffective for people who have a particularly strong aversion to certain scents or smells. Some people are allergic or sensitive to essential oils or fragrances, which can cause skin irritation or other negative reactions.

Finally, it is critical to understand that body odour therapy should not be used in place of medical treatment or professional therapy. While it can be an effective complementary therapy, it is not a replacement for professional medical or psychological care.

Conclusion

Overall, body odour therapy can be a beneficial and natural tool for anxiety management. Individuals can improve their overall well-being and quality of life by using scents and smell to promote relaxation and reduce feelings of anxiety. However, it is critical to recognize the therapy's limitations and to seek professional medical or psychological treatment when necessary.

Chapter 5: Including Body Odour Therapy in Your Wellness Routine

This chapter will look at how people can incorporate body odour therapy into their overall wellness routine. Individuals can reap the full benefits of body odour therapy for anxiety management and relaxation by incorporating it into a regular self-care routine.

Establishing a Self-Care Routine

A self-care routine is a consistent practice of caring for one's physical, emotional, and mental well-being. Individuals can make body odour therapy a regular part of their overall wellness routine by developing a self-care routine that includes it.

Some self-care practices that may include body odour therapy are as follows:

- Taking a bath with essential oils to relax In a quiet space

- use a diffuser with calming scents for meditation or relaxation.
- Applying a personalized scent blend before bedtime to promote better sleep
- To promote a sense of freshness and well-being, wear natural-fiber clothing and use natural deodourants.
- Including Body odour Therapy in the Therapy Session
- Individuals working with a mental health professional can also incorporate body odour therapy into therapy sessions. During therapy sessions, aromatherapy, and custom scent blends can be used to promote relaxation and reduce feelings of anxiety.

Therapists may also recommend using body odour therapy as a tool for anxiety management outside of therapy sessions, such as diffusing calming scents in the home or using a custom scent blend during stressful times.

Individuals can benefit from body odour therapy by incorporating it into their self-care routine and therapy sessions.

Chapter 6: Selecting the Best Scent

Choosing the right scent is critical when using body odour therapy to relieve anxiety. Different scents have different effects on the body and mind, and choosing the right scent can greatly improve the efficacy of this therapy.

Here are some suggestions for selecting the best scent for body odour therapy:

Discover the Effects of Different Scents: Scents can have various effects on the body and mind. Lavender, for example, is known for its calming and relaxing properties, whereas peppermint is invigorating and energizing.

Before choosing a scent for body odour therapy, it can be beneficial to research the effects of various scents and select one that corresponds to your specific needs and goals for this therapy.

Consider Your Preferences: While understanding the effects of various scents is important, personal preferences must also be taken into consideration. If you dislike the scent of lavender, for example, it may not be as effective for body odour therapy.

experiment with various scents: Finding the right scent for body odour therapy may require some trial and error. Begin by experimenting with different scents and observing how your body and mind react to each one.

Create Your Scent Blend: Many people find that making their scent blend is the most effective way to use body odour therapy for anxiety relief. You can create a personalized scent that is tailored to your specific needs and preferences by blending different scents.

Conclusion

Choosing the right scent for anxiety relief is an important part of body odour therapy. You can maximize the effectiveness of this therapy and promote relaxation and well-being by understanding the effects of different scents, considering personal preferences, experimenting with different scents, and customizing your scent blend.

Chapter 7: Body Odour Therapy Risks and Precautions

While body odour therapy can be a safe and effective way to manage anxiety, it is critical to understand the risks and take precautions to ensure that it is used safely and effectively.

Here are some risks and precautions to take when using body odour therapy:

Reactions to allergens: Some people may be allergic to essential oils or fragrance blends. It is critical to perform a patch test on a small area of skin before using a new scent to ensure that no allergic reaction occurs.

Sensitivity or Irritation: Certain essential oils or fragrance blends may cause irritation or sensitivity in some people. If you experience any discomfort, redness, or irritation while using a new scent, stop using it right away.

Pregnancy or medical issues: Some essential oils should not be used during pregnancy or by people who have certain medical conditions. It is critical to consult with a healthcare professional before using any new scent to ensure that it is safe for use.

Essential Oil Quality: Not all essential oils are the same. It is critical to choose high-quality essential oils that are pure and free of synthetic additives when using essential oils for body odour therapy.

Correct Dilution: To avoid skin irritation or sensitivity, essential oils should be properly diluted before use. When using essential oils for body odour therapy, make sure to follow the recommended dilution guidelines.

Conclusion

While body odour therapy can be a safe and effective way to manage anxiety, it is critical to understand the risks and take precautions to ensure that it is used safely and effectively. Individuals can use body odour therapy to promote relaxation and well-being while minimizing potential risks by performing patch tests, using high-quality essential oils, properly diluting essential oils, and consulting with healthcare professionals as needed.

Chapter 8: Conclusion

Body odour therapy can be an effective tool for reducing anxiety while also promoting relaxation and well-being. Individuals can tap into the mind-body connection and promote a sense of calm and inner peace by harnessing the power of scent.

While not for everyone, body odour therapy is a safe and natural alternative to traditional anxiety management techniques. Individuals can use this therapy to improve their overall health and well-being by understanding the link between body odour and emotion, selecting the right scent, and taking the necessary precautions to ensure safety.

Finally, the effectiveness of body odour therapy is determined by the individual. It is critical to approach this therapy with an open mind, to experiment with various scents and techniques, and to be patient with the process. Body odour therapy, with commitment and dedication, can be a valuable addition to any anxiety management regimen.

Resources for further information on body odour therapy

Here are some additional resources for learning more about body odour therapy:

- AromaCulture: This website provides aromatherapy and body odour therapy resources such as articles, courses, and an online community.
- NAHA (National Association for Holistic Aromatherapy): NAHA is a non-profit organisation that promotes the use of

essential oils and aromatherapy in a safe manner. They provide a variety of aromatherapy resources, such as articles, research, and education.

- IJCA (International Journal of Clinical Aromatherapy): IJCA is a peer-reviewed journal devoted to the clinical application of essential oils and aromatherapy. It provides articles and research on a variety of body odour therapy-related topics.

- Robert Tisserand and Rodney Young's Essential Oil Safety is a comprehensive guide to the safe use of essential oils: It discusses the possible risks and precautions associated with using essential oils for body odour therapy.

- Aromatherapy and Subtle Energy Techniques: Joni Keim and Ruah Bull's book Aromatherapy and Subtle Energy Techniques provides a comprehensive guide to the use of essential oils and aromatherapy for emotional and spiritual well-being. It contains information on body odour therapy as well as other novel approaches to aromatherapy.

Individuals can gain a better understanding of body odour therapy and its potential benefits for anxiety management and overall health and wellness by exploring these resources.